vaccines: merits & demerits

VACCINES

Merits & Demerits

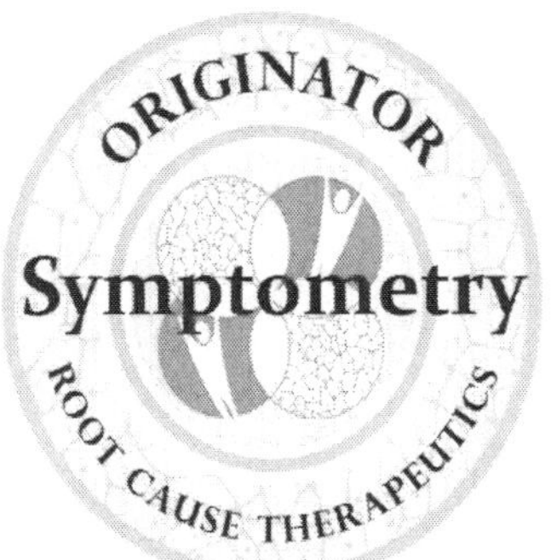

First edition

© Copyright 2011, Symptometry, Inc.

I dedicate this book to all those who continue to find ways to improve vaccination and immunization.

CONTENTS

INTRODUCTION

As recently as 2005, both the residents and chiefs of Kano, North Nigeria, vehemently opposed their government's effort to vaccinate the Kano school children against polio. Was their fear justified? Yes, it was.

The reason their fear was justified was thousands of African children had deformed legs after immunization, especially after the polio immunization. In the United States, thousands of children develop autism, stuttering, dyslexia or complete loss of speech after immunization.

What is most puzzling about the immunization program is that millions of children, globally, don't suffer from the short-term effects of immunization. This makes immunization controversial to some but not so controversial to others.

The purpose of this book is to discuss in great detail the constituents of the vaccines, what can be done to stay healthy without immunization and what should be done on the day of immunization so that the adjuvants in the vaccine do not hurt the immunized person.

CHAPTER ONE
The Sad Beginning

The first doctors who found something fundamentally wrong with vaccines and investigated vaccinosis were not allopathic physicians or MDs as they are now called. They were British homoeopathic physicians. This happened as far back as 1857.

The names of these two British doctors were: Dr. Richard Hughes and Dr. J. Compton Burnett. It was Dr. Burnett who coined the term vaccinosis to mean a "long-lasting morbid state engendered by the vaccine virus implant".

The news that vaccines are the worse antagonists of DNA, after poison, is not an overnight sensation. It has been around for centuries.

Today, many parents are very hesitant when it comes to having their children vaccinated. This is because they have first-hand knowledge of what immunization did to their child or what it did to the child of a person they know.

Is their fear justified? Yes, it is. The question is, if their fear is justified why are governments still insisting that children be immunized? A history lesson will be of some importance at this point.

CHAPTER TWO
History of Vaccination

Infant mortality has been a major public health concern for thousands of years.

Once upon a time, many infants were stillborn. Most of those who made it died shortly after birth due to tetanus and gonorrheal infection during childbirth. The rest hardly celebrated their tenth birthday due to smallpox, diphtheria, pertussis (whooping cough), mumps, rubella or measles.

For thousands of years, the population of the entire continent of Africa and Europe could not reach one million inhabitants.

As a result, no nation could develop a viable work force.

The scientific community did its best to solve this problem but each time scientists tried to find a solution to premature death and infant mortality, they ran out of ideas. The ancient Turks had the answer because they were far ahead of the rest of the world when it came to inoculation.

However, it should be noted that the terms inoculation, immunization, vaccine and vaccination should not be used interchangeably. They are totally different concepts.

A _**vaccine**_ is a man-made product whose sole purpose is to prevent specific microbes from attacking a person. The idea that a vaccine boosts an individual's immune system has not been proven until this day.

Even though it is true that certain vaccines prevent certain infectious diseases, it is also true that vaccines make some immunized individuals more vulnerable to other infectious diseases and to chronic skin conditions such as susceptibility to keloid and warts.

___Inoculation___ has three meanings: 1) it refers to the introduction of a similar microbe into a person who is suffering from a specific infectious disease 2) it refers to the introduction of a live microbe into a healthy person in order to prevent a specific disease and 3) it means permanent protection from the microbe that once caused a disease.

> For instance, a child who had measles and survived will never have measles again. S/he is now naturally ___inoculated___ against the measles virus. The ancient Turks discovered inoculation.

Vaccination specifically refers to the introduction of the cowpox virus into a person who is suffering from smallpox. It also prevents smallpox. Dr. Edward Jenner invented it.

Vaccination derives from the Latin word *vacca* meaning cow. It was public health experts, not microbiologists, who called the process of using a microbe to prevent a specific disease, *vaccination*.

Vaccination is a very limited concept. This was why public health experts coined the term "immunization" to broaden its applicability to the diseases that other microbes cause. Even though the term was broadened, the definition of a vaccine still remains the same (see above).

Immunization refers to a man-made prevention of childhood infectious diseases with a vaccine. Each immunization targets a specific microbe or group of microbes. The microbes that have been targeted so far include mumps, diphtheria, whooping cough virus, tetanus, measles, rubella and polio.

Therefore, immunization is not vaccination. Also, inoculation is not vaccination or immunization.

These days, immunization applies to children, and vaccination applies to adults. For instance, we say senior citizens are being vaccinated (not immunized) against influenza.

CHAPTER THREE
Two Groups of Children

Symptometry discovered that when it comes to resisting diseases, there are two groups of children: 1) breastfed children and 2) non-breastfed children.

Then, there are other factors that determine how a child will react to immunization. The two most predominant factors are: 1) the health of the child on the day of immunization and 2) the food the child eats on the day of immunization.

Experience has shown that a child who was immunized when s/he was still coughing, having runny nose and fatigued eyes, was most likely to react more violently to the vaccine than the healthier child.

Experience has also shown that breastfed children who didn't eat boiled egg, didn't drink apple juice or orange juice or didn't eat an apple on the day of the immunization were able to maintain their health after the immunization.

The heaviest casualties of immunization continue to be:
1) enzyme-deficient children who were not breastfed but ate boiled egg, an apple or drank apple juice or orange juice on the day of immunization
2) enzyme-deficient children who were breastfed but ate boiled egg, an apple or banana, or either drank apple juice or orange juice on the day of immunization and
3) children who were sick on the day of the immunization.

CHAPTER FOUR
Contribution of Ancient Turks

The Turks learned centuries ago that the microbe in a diseased person would protect a healthy person from the infectious disease that made the person sick.

This knowledge was passed on from generation to generation. Even though modernity is making this ancient tradition obsolete, many Turkish grandparents and traditionalists are still holding on to its strands.

Some individuals in Medieval Europe got wind of this Turkish cultural practice and they tried it in Germany, in France and in England.

For instance, in 1718, Lady Mary Montagu inoculated her children against smallpox, Jensen of Germany did likewise in 1770, Mrs. Sevel of Germany did it in 1772, Benjamin Jesty of England did it in 1774, Rendall of England did it in 1782 and in 1791 Peter Plett of Germany did it in 1791.

They all had fantastic results.

Confident of the idea that inoculation works, Dr. Edward Jenner, a British physician and bacteriologist used the cowpox virus to vaccinate children against smallpox in 1798. He did not call it inoculation because his product came from a cow.

Around the same year, 1798, Dr. Samuel Hahnemann also lunched homoeopathy.

It is not clear whether both got the same idea from inoculation, but what is known is that they produced totally different therapeutic products.

CHAPTER FIVE
The Approach of Dr. Samuel Hahnemann

Dr. Hahnemann produced homoeopathic remedies and Dr. Jenner produced the first vaccine from cowpox.

The pillar of Dr. Hahnemann's homoeopathy was *similia similibus curantur* meaning, "let likes cure likes". The concept was extended to the assumption that smallpox will cure smallpox.

Likwise, malaria will cure hereditary malaria and it will also prevent contemporary malaria; cancer will cure both hereditary cancer and contemporary cancer; diabetes will cure hereditary diabetes and prevent contemporary diabetes; tuberculosis will cure hereditary tuberculosis and it will also prevent hereditary tuberculosis, and so on and so forth.

Instead of experimenting with inoculation, Dr. Hahnemann experimented with cinchona, the bark of the tree that Peruvians used to treat malaria.

Then, he applied his concept of letting likes cure likes to the product that would stimulate, in a healthy person, symptoms that are similar to those of a sick person who is suffering from a particular disease.

Dr. Hahnemann's interpretation of letting likes cure likes did not sit well with some homoeopaths who felt that he had deviated from the original paradigm.

After a few years of practice, a few homoeopathic researchers reverted back to the idea of letting likes cure likes by producing remedies with the fluid from people who were suffering from all kinds of diseases.

They called their remedies *sarcodes* and *nosodes*. It should be stated for the record that Dr. Hahnemann never produced sarcodes and nosodes. He only produced remedies from plants and from a few minerals.

The detractors and critics of homoeopathy thought homoeopaths were insane by making remedies out of diseased tissues. They were not insane. They knew something that many intellectuals did not know. These homoeopaths became more successful at curing diseases than Dr. Hahnemann who founded homoeopathy.

More importantly, they were healthier than their detractors.

They knew that _**where the disease is, there is the remedy**_. Instead of pursuing this idea to the very end and staying the course, some homoeopathic scholars mooted and institutionalized crazy ideas such as drug pictures, the doctrine of signatures, repertorization, etc.

Repertorization muddied the waters to where post-Hahnemann homoeopaths became and are still totally confused. Repertorization remains the Achilles' heel that continues to tarnish the repute of homoeopathy until this day. It is illogical and totally unscientific.

CHAPTER SIX
The Jenner Predicament

Dr. Edward Jenner also faced a very serious problem, especially after many children had been vaccinated.

Even though the children who were vaccinated did not have smallpox, the vaccination created other very serious health problems.

The new condition it created was called _vaccinosis_ (health complications resulting from vaccination). Most, if not all the children who were vaccinated had fever, diarrhea, joint pain, headaches, weakness, nightmares, and many other ailments. Some were so sick that they could not go to school.

The London board of health had to suspend vaccination pending the review of the vaccination process as well as the entire process of vaccine manufacturing. Other districts took similar action.

Bacteriologists who examined the blood of the sick children discovered many other microbes in it. It became apparent that even though the smallpox vaccine protected the children from smallpox, it degraded tissues to the point where other microbes thrived.

Also, it was discovered that the vaccine further weakened the child's immune system.

In order to save vaccination, scientists came up with the idea of replacing the live smallpox virus with an attenuated (weak) virus. This was done but they encountered another problem that was bigger than the first one: how to preserve the vaccine so that it does not deteriorate.

CHAPTER SEVEN
Vaccine Preservative Nightmare

Mercury was the first metal that came to mind when scientists thought of preserving the vaccines that had to be produced on a large scale.

Vaccine manufacturers made thimerosal (mercury) the main vaccine preservative for over 200 years until the United Sates government banned it from pediatric vaccines in 1996.

Unfortunately, it was too late. Thimerosal had already ruined millions of lives, worldwide, between 1800 and 1996. It was banned because there was verifiable evidence that it caused the disease that the vaccine was supposed to prevent.

For instance, the polio vaccine caused polio, the mumps vaccine caused mumps, and the measles vaccine caused chickenpox or shingles and so on.

The main advantage of the immunization program was that it significantly reduced infant mortality. As a matter of fact, immunization reduced infant mortality so well that, despite the periodic epidemics of dysentery, influenza, cholera and typhoid, the world's population increased by several billion inhabitants.

However, the largest disadvantage of immunization continues to be the fact that it makes the immunized person vulnerable to other infectious diseases. This is because it targets only a few viruses and bacteria.

In targeting these specific viruses and bacteria, it makes the vaccinated person vulnerable to other microbial attacks.

Finally, its preservatives create a permanent morbidity in the vaccinated person. What is morbidity?

CHAPTER EIGHT
Vaccine Morbidity

Morbidity is a condition that overburdens and weakens DNA to the point where it can no longer transcribe genetic material to RNA (ribonucleic acid). Then, the heavy metals especially aluminum (in children and adult vaccines) and mercury (only in adult vaccines) will denature a person's enzymes.

Nothing in the human body can be produced without enzymatic reaction. If enzymes are being constantly denatured, a person will not be able to produce many proteins.

Also, s/he will not be able to digest many foods. This will cause chronic food allergies. Many children cannot digest milk, greens, fruits, gluten in rice and wheat and so on because of these enzymatic disorders. Let me cite other instances to show how enzyme denaturing can affect a person's immune system.

In the red bone marrow, there are 3 mechanisms: 1) leucopoietic mechanism 2) erythropoietic mechanism and 3) the platelet-producing mechanism.

If the leucopoietic mechanism is impacted because of enzymatic disorders, the person will produce weak T cells or s/he will produce an inadequate number of white blood cells. It is the weak T cells that will make a vaccinated person vulnerable to influenza, chickenpox, hepatitis, malaria, infectious mononucleosis, HIV, viral pneumonia, and so on.

If the platelet mechanism is affected, the person will produce an inadequate number of platelets. Hemophilia occurs in individuals who have an impacted platelet mechanism.

If the erythropoietic mechanism is affected, the person will not be able to produce an adequate number of red blood cells or hemoglobin. This will cause chronic anemia.

Thalassemia or microcystic anemia is the kind of anemia where the person's red blood cells are too small. In macrocystic anemia, the person's red blood cells are bigger than normal.

Sickle cell anemia is the kind of anemia where the person's red blood cells are deformed. People who were not immunized and did not take quinine derivatives don't have sickle cell anemia or its trait.

If, after immunization, the speech mechanism is affected, the person may stutter or s/he may lose h/her ability to speak. If the auditory nerve is affected, the child could be deaf.

If the sphincter vescicae is affected the person will suffer from chronic bed-wetting.

If the skin is affected, the person will develop a very unhealthy skin (skin rash, keloid or succession of boils).

If the kidneys are affected, the person will develop weak kidneys.

Morbidity will plague the immunized person throughout h/her life unless the preservative is neutralized. What is in the vaccine?

CHAPTER NINE
Constituents of Vaccines

According to the CDC (Centers for Disease control and prevention), vaccine additives include:

- Suspending fluid (salt water, distilled water or fluids containing protein)

- Preservatives that help the vaccine to remain unchanged for a certain period of time. They include: phenols, albumin and glycine.

- Adjuvants that serve as vaccine enhancers. They help the vaccine to become very effective against the target.

  Common adjuvants include: aluminum salts (aluminum hydroxide that is also found in antacids, aluminum hydroxyl-phosphate sulfate, aluminum acetate, aluminum phosphate, aluminum potassium sulfate, etc.)

- Hydrochloric acid as a pH stabilizer

- MSG (monosodium glutamate) as a stabilizer. It is a long-term health disruptor that may cause digestive problems It is also in magi cube and in some Oriental cuisines

- Potassium chloride as the adjuster of pH toxicity

- Antibiotics such as streptomycin and neomycin

- Sorbitol as a stabilizer. Sorbitol is sugar.

- Yeast protein. Yeast is a long-term health disruptor. It blooms only when the person's immune system has hit rock bottom.

  It is at this time that it may predispose a person to candidiasis (yeast infection), stomatitis that is popularly known as thrush, fungus around fingernails, fungus in the lungs, in the heart, etc.

- Formaldehyde. Formaldehyde that predisposes the vaccinated person to asthma and to respiratory diseases. This was proven after the Katrina hurricane.

  In the aftermath of this hurricane, most occupants of the temporary housing trailers – which used formaldehyde was used as insulating material - succumbed to asthma and to other respiratory diseases. There was a Congressional hearing on this matter.

What else do the vaccine additives do?

Aluminum hydroxide will cause chronic constipation or severe abdominal pains. *Aluminum phosphate* is corrosive to tissue and *aluminum sulfate* will cause chronic acne or boils in susceptible individuals.

It is aluminum phosphate that makes people susceptible to all kinds of ulcers and it is *aluminum acetate* that makes people to develop skin rashes or an unhealthy skin.

Aluminum hydroxide is insoluble in water. Since the human body is 94% water, aluminum hydroxide will remain a permanent nutrient blocker and process inhibitor in the vaccinated person.

Every person who suffers from Alzheimer's disease has a lot of aluminum deposits in h/her brain. Also, most Alzheimer's patients were vaccinated as adults.

Let me at this point discuss how aluminum hydroxide makes a person susceptible to dyslexia, color blindness and autism.

CHAPTER TEN
Dyslexia and Color blindness

Dyslexia is the condition where a person cannot read because letters are running together. In color blindness, the person cannot properly contrast or distinguish colors.

The genes in the various segments of the retina must have nutrients in order to produce the various chemicals to distinguish colors and to facilitate reading.

In a few individuals in whom aluminum hydroxide is blocking nutrient intake into the cells of the retina, their eye disorder cannot be cured unless the aluminum salt has been ionized.

Russian roulette

At some point, every person will be sickened by immunization or vaccination. Some will suffer from its short-term consequences. Others will suffer from its long-term consequences.

The term Russian roulette is a term that Symptometry uses to characterize immunization/vaccination. This is because nobody knows exactly the kind of disease s/he will get from immunization or from vaccination in the short run or in the long run.

S/he could suffer from enzymatic disorders, constipation, colic, dyslexia, color blindness, stuttering or myopia, unhealthy skin and dry skin. This list goes on.

CHAPTER ELEVEN
Immunization and Autism

Aluminum hydroxide is worse when the pH is off balance. This happens when the person eats boiled egg, a banana, an orange or an apple or s/he drinks lemonade, apple juice or orange juice on the day of vaccination.

Boiled egg or hominy will cause alkalosis. Then, banana, orange, lemonade, apple, apple juice and orange juice will cause acidosis. All the pH adjusters in the vaccine will be totally useless during alkalosis and acidosis.

Alkalosis and acidosis are situations where nerves, especially the brain nerves become too sluggish when they are sending or receiving signals.

This is because blood has become too acidic or too alkaline. Sluggishness of brain signals will affect comprehension, learning, calculation, creativity, judging distance, etc.

During alkalosis and acidosis, aluminum hydroxide will prevent the production of many brain peptides by shutting down the peptide production process in the brain. It is the shutting down of the peptide production process that will set the stage for autism.

If the following acid or alkaline foods are served in the morning prior to immunization, they could predispose a person to autism: apples, apple juice, orange, orange juice, banana, boiled eggs and lemonade.

The food that the child is fed on the day of immunization will determine whether s/he will weather the immunization or s/he will be adversely affected by it.

Millions of children are being immunized throughout the world every year. It is only the children who are sick prior to the immunization, and children who either suffered from acidosis or from alkalosis before they were immunized who would end up suffering from the immediate effects of vaccination.

This is where an apple may help. Apples are tricky fruits. If they are organic, their skin will not have wax but if they are not organic, their skin will be waxed. Wax is a nutrient blocker.

Then, apple has valeric acid, malic acid and salicylates. I will recommend that the *apple be eaten at least 24 hours after the immunization* but not on the day of immunization.

CHAPTER TWELVE
Effects of Vaccines

Immunization has short-term and long-term consequences. Every person who was immunized will suffer from the long-term effect of the vaccine.

This is because the _principle of atomic conductivity_ circulates the tiniest drop of the adjuvants and the vaccine preservatives throughout the person's body. Then, the adjuvants and the preservatives will become a burden on DNA.

Parents complained for decades that vaccination made their children autistic. However, as is often the case, the United

States federal government wanted more evidence of this linkage.

It was only after the link between immunization and autism was firmly established that the federal government, in 1980, set up a fund called _National Vaccine Injury Compensation Program_ to compensate the families of autistic children.

This program is an acknowledgement of the fact that even though vaccines have considerably reduced infant mortality; they continue to be a long-term health hazard.

So many children are in special education class because of the ill effects of immunization, fetal alcohol syndrome, and drug injury during gestation or brain injury during childbirth.

CHAPTER THIRTEEN
Symptoms of Autism

An autistic child suffers from a very weak memory, inadequate intellect, withdrawn personality or hyperactivity.

Then, if the home and school environments are not conducive to h/her harmonious growth and development, the autistic child will develop additional neurological disorders.

An autistic child who is not able to perform in class and who wets the bed almost every day will begin to suffer from low self-esteem.

Low self-esteem could lead to total withdrawal or to hyperactivity. Then, withdrawal or hyperactivity will, sooner or later, lead to depression, irritability or violent temper.

Depression will become more severe in the child who lacks nurturing and attention. Many autistic children develop exceptional talents as a way of compensating for their other inadequacies. What is nurturing?

Nurturing

Nurturing is the sum total of actions that bring the best out of a person. For example, hugging, greeting the child with enthusiasm, kissing appropriately, touching appropriately, praising the child after a job has been well done, combing h/her hair, and helping the child to do h/her homework, are acts of nurturing.

CHAPTER FOURTEEN
Living *without* Vaccinations

Many parents don't vaccinate their children and themselves. They take vitamin C supplements, lysine, arginine, glycine and zinc on a regular basis to prevent microbes from causing an infection.

Then, there are parents who don't take any special measures to protect their children from microbes other than good breast-feeding.

I personally know a family that does not vaccinate their children for religious reasons. Their children are now teenagers and they are healthier than most children who were immunized.

Here is what many people are not aware of. Good breast-feeding lasting for at least six months, not eating citrus fruits, good hygiene and sanitation and not eating rye bread constitute the natural way of building a strong immune system.

In 1798, Dr. Edward Jenner did not study the effect that good breast-feeding had on children. Also, he did not study the effects of nurturing, good hygiene and sanitation on health. If he did, he would have come to a totally different conclusion with regard to weak immunity.

As I mentioned earlier, the Turks inoculated themselves with the fluid from the sick person.

Even though vaccines have many disadvantages, they have been helpful when people know what to do before and after taking them. People who take supplements may all not be successful at *preventing* microbes from hurting them as the Turks were. Here is why.

Some microbes feed off vitamins and amino acids. Then, drinking a beverage that has **_citric acid_** will prevent zinc from getting into the thymus gland and into the red bone marrow. T cells cannot mature if the thymus gland can't get zinc to produce the enzymes that will speed up their maturity.

It is for the above reason that Symptometry will not recommend that people take matters into their own hand and self-medicate. If some parents don't want their children to be immunized, Symptometry is ready to properly guide them in achieving their objective.

Microbes get their growth factors from tattered cells, not from the blood stream.

Therefore, a person who lacks the proper knowledge about how to strengthen h/her immune system will end up weakening it.

CHAPTER FIFTEEN
Necessity of Vaccines

Vaccines are necessary for individuals who count on the government to protect them or their children from microbes.

Governments want to have a healthy work force and healthy children. This is why they are right in protecting vulnerable people who don't have a clue about what to do to be healthy.

As I mentioned earlier, I know a family that does not subscribe to immunization. Are their children dead? No, they are not. They are all alive and healthy. There millions of such families across the globe.

If a person knows what to do to strengthen h/her child's immune system, nothing should prevent h/her from applying h/her brilliant preventive knowledge.

Symptometry, which is the just, the right, the scientific, the natural and the logical way to make a person healthy, is backing the effort of knowledgeable individuals in matters of health.

The family I was talking about is now benefiting from the expertise of Symptometry. They have finally found what they have been looking for: an excellent frame of reference in matters of health. Symptometry is that frame of reference.

People who know how to make their cells divide or know a doctor who knows how to do it, will never produce **_growth factors for microbes_**. It is these individuals who will have a robust immune system.

Also, people who benefit from nurturing will have a very strong immune system. A person who has a strong immune system will not need vaccination or immunization.

Symptometry neutralizes the additives, the adjuvants and the heavy metals in vaccines through **_ionization_**. This is how it keeps vaccinated people healthy in the short term as well as in the long term.

INDEX

ABOUT THE AUTHOR

Dr. Maxwell Nartey is DHM (Doctor of Homoeopathic Medicine), NHD (Doctor of Natural Health), Fellow of the British Institute of Homoeopathy, founder of the American College of Symptometry and lecturer of Symptometry.

He is a published author and a regular contributor to the Anita L. Collins "My Childrens' Children" (sic) radio talk show on WGNU 920AM , St. Louis, Missouri.

He has extensively researched vaccines and he is now ionizing, through Symptometry, the morbidity of vaccines so that people will be healthier. The ionization of the adjuvants of vaccines has proven to be a phenomenal success.

ORIGINATOR
Symptometry
ROOT CAUSE THERAPEUTICS

9456362R0004

Made in the USA
Charleston, SC
14 September 2011